The Long and Healthy Life of the Chinese: Exploring Cultural Traditions for Health and Wellness

INDEX

Introduction

In this book, we will explore the lifestyle of the Chinese and how it contributes to their longevity. China is known for having one of the longest-lived populations in the world, with many inhabitants reaching 100 years of age and beyond. The longevity of the Chinese is a very interesting and complex topic, which depends on a combination of factors, including lifestyle, diet and genetics.

In general, the Chinese have a longer life expectancy than other nations, averaging about 77 years for men and 83 years for women.

Today we will explore the food habits, traditional medical practices and cultural traditions that impact the health and longevity of the Chinese.

Chapter 1

The Chinese Diet - The Key to Longevity

Nutrition is a crucial element in Chinese culture and plays a fundamental role in their longevity and well-being. Chinese dietary philosophy is based on the concept of balance, which is expressed both in the variety of foods and in their preparation.

In China, nutrition is seen as a means of maintaining health and prevent disease, rather than as a simple source of nourishment for the body. Chinese cuisine is famous for its ability to combine different ingredients to create nutritionally balanced dishes.

Chinese cuisine follows the philosophy of balancing yin and yang, which represent the two opposing forces of cold and heat, humidity and dryness, sweetness and bitterness. For example, efforts are made to balance vegetables and proteins, such as meat or tofu, to create a well-balanced, complete meal.

The ingredients used in Chinese cuisine are often natural or not processed, such as fresh vegetables, meat and fish, and the Chinese diet limits the use of fats and sugars. Instead, large amounts of whole grains, fruits and vegetables are favored to ensure a balanced and healthy diet.

Furthermore, Chinese cuisine also takes advantage of the medicinal properties of herbs and spices, using them to treat specific ailments. For example, garlic is used to lower blood pressure, while ginger is used to reduce nausea and vomiting.

Food preparation in China is an art, requiring attention to detail and the quality of ingredients.

For example, foods are often boiled orjumped to preserve its nutritional value.

In addition, Chinese culture promotes a moderate lifestyle and a balanced diet, avoiding overeating and being overweight. This approach to nutrition is an important factor in the longevity and health of the Chinese population.

In summary, the Chinese diet represents a combination of balance, variety, natural ingredients and artisanal preparation of food, which plays a fundamental role in the health and longevity of the Chinese population and which consequently is an essential element.

Chapter 2

The importance of physical activity in daily life

Regular physical activity has multiple benefits, such as helping maintain health and longevity. It also helps reduce stress and anxiety, improve blood circulation, increase muscle strength and flexibility, maintain a healthy weight, and help prevent numerous chronic diseases, including cardiovascular disease, diabetes, and depression.

Tai Chi, in particular, is an example of a physical exercise that has multiple benefits: it helps improve physical health, it helps improve concentration, balance and coordination. In addition, the meditation that accompanies the Tai Chi movements helps reduce stress and improve mental health.

Walking or taking long walks is another form of physical activity that is accessible and healthy for all ages. Walking helps maintain good blood circulation, improve joint health and prevent chronic diseases such as diabetes and cardiovascular disease. In addition, walking outdoors in nature also has a positive effect on mental well-being, as it helps reduce stress and anxiety.

Gymnastics and dance are other forms of exercise that combine exercise with enjoyment. Gymnastics helps improve muscle strength and flexibility, while dance helps improve balance and coordination. Furthermore, gymnastics and dancing are also a great opportunity to socialize and make new friends.

In summary, regular physical activity is an important factor in the longevity and health of the Chinese population. The practice of traditional physical exercises such as Tai Chi, walking, gymnastics and dance helps maintain an active and healthy lifestyle, which has multiple positive benefits for physical and mental health. It is important to encourage and support regular physical activity as an important part of daily life to reap the maximum health benefits.

Chapter 3

Healing with Ancient Wisdom - The Traditional Medical Practices of Chinese Medicine

Traditional Chinese Medicine (TCM) is a medical system that dates back thousands of years and is based on a unique understanding of human nature and the world around us. TCM considers the human body as a collection of interconnected organs and systems and believes that the energy balance between these elements is crucial for health and disease prevention.

TCM differs from Western medicines in that it focuses on treating the root causes of disease rather than treating the symptoms. For example, instead of just treating the symptoms of a disease, TCM seeks to understand why the body is reacting the way it does and to correct the root problem.

To maintain and restore energy balance, TCM uses a variety of techniques and therapies, including moxibustion, acupuncture, TUI NA massage, the use of medicinal herbs, and exercises such as Tai Chi and Qigong. These techniques are used individually or in combination to create a personalized treatment for each individual, taking into account his uniqueness and individual needs.

Traditional Chinese Medicine is still very popular in China and around the world, and continues to be studied and practiced by many people who are looking for a natural way to maintain and improve their health. Despite its differences from Western medicines, TCM is recognized as an effective and well-developed medical system with a long history of success in the prevention and treatment of disease.

Chapter 4

Chinese moxibustion: History, technique and benefits of its applications in traditional medicine

Moxibustion is a technique that is part of traditional Chinese medicine and dates back to more than 2000 years ago. Its origin is uncertain, but some historical writings suggest that it was originally used to treat disease and pain.

Basically, moxibustion consists of using heat to stimulate certain points on the body, which are considered important for the circulation of Qi (vital energy) according to traditional Chinese medicine, to warm the skin and underlying tissues, which help promote blood circulation and reduce pain.

This warmth is produced using a mugwort candle, known as a "moxa," which is lit and placed near or directly on the skin.

Moxibustion is used to treat a range of conditions, including headaches, joint pain, sleep disturbances and female health issues. Also, it comes used to strengthen the immune system and improve digestive function.

Typically, moxibustion is performed by a skilled practitioner who places moxa on the skin and lets it burn for a set amount of time. The technique is generally safe and non-invasive, and many patients report feeling more relaxed and invigorated after the session.

However, it is not a universally accepted form of medical treatment and has not been scientifically proven to be effective for treating all conditions for which it is used. There are also some precautions from take, how to avoid using moxibustion in areas where there is skin disease or inflammation, or in the presence of some chronic conditions.

Furthermore, moxibustion should only be practiced by experienced professionals who have the appropriate training in this technique and who are able to evaluate the safety of the patient and any contraindications.

Despite this, many patients report that they have benefited from moxibustion and have experienced improvements in their health and quality of life.

However, it is important to speak to your doctor before starting any form of alternative treatment, including moxibustion, to evaluate the safety and effectiveness based on your individual health condition.

Chapter 5

The Art of Acupuncture: Understanding and Experience Traditional Chinese Medicine

Acupuncture is an ancient medical practice dating back more than 2,000 years and stemming from it from traditional Chinese medicine.

It is based on the theory that the flow of vital energy (known as "Qi" or "Chi") through the human body is influenced by a series of specific points along the energy meridians. These points are accessible through the skin and are used to treat a wide range of ailments and health conditions.

Acupuncture is a safe and effective technique for treating many diseases and conditions. Numerous studies have demonstrated its effectiveness in reducing pain, improving blood circulation and reducing stress and anxiety.

Additionally, acupuncture has been used successfully to treat a variety of ailments, including headaches, muscle and joint pain, depression, anxiety, insomnia, digestive and menstrual problems, and so much more.

During an acupuncture session, needles are inserted into specific areas of the body where acupuncture points are located. These needles can be left in place for 15-30 minutes or even longer, depending on the severity of the ailment and the patient's individual needs. Most patients report feeling relaxed during the session and perceiving an improvement in symptoms.

The safety of acupuncture is very high, as the needles used are thin and disposable, which reduces the risk of infections. Furthermore, Acupuncture is a non-invasive technique that has no effects negative side effects when performed properly by a qualified practitioner.

If you are looking for a non-invasive and safe option to treat your health problems, Acupuncture may be a good option for you to consider. I recommend you speak to a qualified professional for
determine if this healing technique is right for your individual needs.

Chapter 6

The regenerating power of Tui Na

Tui Na Massage is a traditional Chinese healing technique that involves massaging and manipulating the muscles and tissues of the body. This type of massage uses compression, stretching, and percussion techniques tissue manipulation to help improve blood circulation blood, reduce pain and increase flexibility.

Tui Na is also used in cases of muscle and joint pain, ache head, digestive disorders and female health problems.

During a Tui Na Massage session, the practitioner uses the hands, elbows, knees and feet to manipulate the body's tissues and promote blood circulation. Typically, the massage is done on a massage table, but it can also be done in a chair or on the floor.

In summary, Tui Na Massage is an important healing technique traditional Chinese tea that offers many health and wellness benefits. This ancient technique still stands widely practiced in China and around the world, and continues to be an important tool for health care and well-being.

Tui Na Massage, in addition to being used to treat the health problems mentioned, also has many other therapeutic properties. For example, it helps relax tense muscles, improve joint mobility, and reduce stress and anxiety.

Additionally, Tui Na Massage is often combined with other traditional Chinese healing techniques, such as Acupuncture and Moxibustion, for a even more powerful effect. This type of integration of different traditional Chinese healing techniques is called (as already mentioned) "TCM" or "Traditional Chinese Medicine".

Tui Na Massage is safe, and is performed by experienced

practitioners who have completed appropriate training and are proficient in massage techniques. Before a Tui Na Massage session, the practitioner can assess the patient's condition and adapt massage techniques to meet your specific needs.

Chapter 7

The balance of Tai Chi: discover the ancient Chinese martial art for health and longevity

Tai Chi is an ancient and profound practice that derives from traditional Chinese medicine. Also known as "Tai Chi Chuan," this system of exercises comprises a series of slow, flowing movements performed in coordination with breathing and mental focus.

Tai Chi was originally developed as a martial art, but has been adapted in recent centuries to become a form of exercise and meditation.

This practice is now widely used as a means to improve health and well-being, and is practiced by people of all ages and fitness levels.

One of Tai Chi's biggest benefits is that it is a low-impact activity that can be performed by people of all ages and with a wide range of health conditions. Helps improve flexibility, strength, balance and coordination.

Tai Chi is often described as a form of moving meditation, requiring intense concentration on breathing and body movements.

This type of focus helps improve body awareness and promote a greater sense of peace and well-being.

Furthermore, it is a social practice that is often performed in groups, which helps create a sense of community and improve interpersonal relationships. This type of social interaction can be especially helpful for older people who live alone or who need more social support.
As a practice accessible to anyone, it continues to be an important part of Chinese cultural tradition.

Chapter 8

The Power of Qigong: Explore the ancient Chinese art of breathing and movement

Qigong is an ancient practice that derives from traditional Chinese medicine and includes a series of breathing, movement and exercises meditation.

The word "Qigong" literally means "working with life energy" and this practice is used to improve health and longevity.

Qigong encompasses a wide range of techniques and styles, but in general, the exercises are slow and fluid, and include body movements, deep breathing, and meditation. This practice helps improve the circulation of blood and chi or vital energy in the body, and is often used as a means to reduce stress and improve sleep quality.

One of the major advantages of Qigong is that it is an activity that can be performed by 18-year-olds up to the elderly person of 70/80 years. Additionally, Qigong is a form of moving meditation that helps improve body awareness and promote a greater sense of peace and well-being.

Qigong is often practiced as a form of self-care, but it's also used in conjunction with traditional Chinese medicine, such as acupuncture, to treat health conditions, including chronic pain, insomnia, and chronic disease.

In addition to its many health benefits, Qigong is also considered a spiritual art that aims to promote inner balance and a heightened awareness of one's connection to the universe. Through regular Qigong practice, one develops a greater awareness of one's physical and mental health, and one can experience greater inner peace and an increased ability to manage stress.

Additionally, Qigong is often performed outdoors, in natural areas such as parks or gardens, which helps create a connection with nature and promote a feeling of peace and harmony with one's surroundings.

Finally, Qigong is an accessible practice and can be easily learned by anyone, regardless of fitness level or flexibility. There are many Qigong teachers and classes available, and there are also many online resources and books that can help you learn the movements and technique.

In summary, Qigong is an ancient practice that offers many benefits to the health and well-being, and which can be learned by anyone.

This practice certainly deserves to be considered as an option for whom look for a way to improve their health and life.

Chapter 9

Meditation in Chinese medicine

Meditation is an ancient practice that has been integrated into many cultures and traditions, including the Chinese one. Meditation has been used to improve mental and physical health and to increase awareness of self and the world around us.

In Chinese culture, meditation has traditionally been seen as a way to achieve balance between the body and mind and to promote longevity. Practicing this technique helps reduce stress, increase concentration and improve the quality of sleep, all of which can help increase longevity.

Furthermore, this has also been associated with other health benefits such as reduced risk of cardiovascular disease, lower blood pressure and a stronger immune system.

Chapter 10

Self-massage therapy

Self-massage therapy is a common practice in traditional Chinese medicine. This technique involves hand massaging certain areas of the body to improve blood circulation and joint flexibility, as well as promote overall health.

Massage has long been used in China to treat a variety of ailments such as: headache, muscle and joint pain, insomnia and fatigue.

There are several Chinese
self-massage techniques, including
leg, abdomen, head and ear massage.
Each technique is performed in a
specific way to help treat specific
problems and improve overall health.

Self-massage therapy can be a great
addition to a balanced, healthy lifestyle
and can help improve health and
vitality.

THE MERIDIANS OF THE (MTC)

1. **Heart Meridian (Xin):** Associated with the heart and circulatory system, this meridian is responsible for blood circulation and temperature regulation of the body.

2. **Small Intestine Meridian (Dai):**associated with the small intestine, this meridian is responsible for the digestion and assimilation of nutrients.

3. **Stomach Meridian (Wei):**Associated with the stomach, this meridian is responsible for digestion and the circulation of Qi.

4. **Spleen Meridian (Pi):** associated with the spleen, this meridian is responsible for digestion, assimilation of nutrients and physical energy.

5. **Liver Meridian (Gan):** Associated with the liver, this meridian is responsible for regulating the flow of Qi and blood circulation.

6. **Lung Meridian (Fei):**associated with the lungs, this meridian is responsible for breathing and regulating vital energy.

7. **Bladder Meridian (Pang Guang)**:associated with the bladder, this meridian is responsible for eliminating toxins and controlling excretory functions.

8. **Gall Bladder Meridian (Dan)**:associated with the gallbladder, this meridian is responsible for digestion, the regulation of bile and the regulation of vital energy.

9. **Ren meridian (Shen):**associated with the kidneys, this meridian is responsible for regulating blood production, hormonal balance and vital energy.

10. **Triple Warmer Meridian (San Jiao):** associated with the triple warmer, this meridian is responsible for controlling body temperature and regulating vital energy.

11. **Pericardium Meridian (Xin Bao):**Associated with the pericardium, this meridian is responsible for blood circulation and heart regulation.

Today I will focus only on 5 of them:

THE KIDNEY MERIDIAN

The Kidney Meridian is one of the 12 major meridians in Traditional Chinese Medicine (TCM). Each of these meridians is associated with a specific organ or organic system and has a precise path in the body.

In TCM, the kidney is considered a very important organ for overall health, as it is associated with vitality, strength and energy. Kidney Meridian Self-Massage Therapy is a way to stimulate and strengthen this organ, as well as to improve health in general.

The Kidney Meridian self-massage technique involves massaging certain areas of the body that are associated with this meridian, such as the knees, thighs, and lower back. These areas are massaged with the hands or a small tool such as a wooden stick or massager, using circular or pressing motions.

Kidney Meridian Self-Massage Therapy has several benefits

health benefits, including increased energy and vitality, a stronger immune system, reduced stress, and improved sleep quality.

THE SPLEEN MERIDIAN

The spleen is an important organ in TCM, as it is associated with digestion, assimilation of food and physical energy. Spleen meridian self-massage therapy is one way to stimulate and strengthen this organ, as well as improve health.

The technique of self-massage of the spleen meridian consists in massage certain areas of the body that are associated with this meridian, such as the stomach region and the lateral rib area.

Spleen meridian self-massage therapy has brought about several health outcomes: improved digestion, increased physical energy, a stronger immune system, and reduced stress.

THE MERIDIAN OF THE HEART

According to traditional Chinese medicine, the heart is considered the governing center of the body, responsible for circulating blood, regulating temperature, and maintaining emotional stability.

The Heart Meridian is also associated with the Shen, or spirit mind, and is considered the most important meridian for mental and emotional health.

Dysfunctions of the heart meridian can cause symptoms such as insomnia, palpitations, anxiety, depression and other emotional disorders.

Treatment of the Heart Meridian may involve the use of techniques such as moxibustion, acupuncture, meditation, and the practice of Qigong and breathing exercises.

It is important to know that the health of the heart meridian is influenced by many factors, including lifestyle, nutrition, exercise and sleep quality. Hence, maintaining a balanced and healthy life, which includes a balanced diet and regular physical activity, can help promote heart meridian health and improve your health.

THE PERICARDIAL MERIDIAN

According to traditional Chinese medicine, the pericardium plays an important role in maintaining balance between the heart and the nervous system. It is considered to be an important regulator of emotions, helping to maintain mental and emotional calm and stability.

If you have problems with the pericardial meridian, these can cause symptoms such as anxiety, irritability,insomnia and other emotional disorders. Therefore it is very important to know that in some cases, the use of techniques such as Moxibustion, Acupuncture, meditation and the practice of breathing exercises and Qigong may be required.

TRIPLE HEATER MERIDIAN

It is associated with a set of organs including the stomach, pancreas and large intestine.

According to traditional Chinese medicine, the triple heater plays an important role in digestion, nutrient absorption and metabolism regulation. It is also associated with body temperature regulation and immune function.

Malfunctions of the Triple Warmer meridian can lead to problems such as: slow digestion, diarrhea, constipation and other digestive disorders.

Chapter 11

Acupressure: healing through the pressure of acupuncture points

Acupressure is a form of alternative therapy used in traditional Chinese medicine that aims to improve health and well-being through the stimulation of specific points on the body.

These points are known as acupuncture points and are located along the meridians, or energy channels, of the body.

Acupressure is similar to acupuncture, but unlike acupuncture which uses needles to stimulate points, acupressure uses manual pressure with your fingers or a tool. The technique consists of gently pressing and massaging the acupuncture points to stimulate the circulation of Qi or as already mentioned earlier, (vital energy), and improve the flow of meridians.

Acupressure is used to treat a wide range of conditions, including chronic pain, digestive disorders, insomnia, stress and anxiety. The therapy can be used alone or in combination with other techniques, such as Acupuncture or Moxibustion, to achieve maximum benefits.

Acupressure is considered safe and free from side effects, but it is important that it is performed by a trained practitioner to avoid complications. Therapy can be customized to meet each person's specific needs and can be adapted over time as conditions change.

Chapter 12

Living in Harmony with the Environment:

How Nature Affects Longevity and Health

The environment in which one lives can significantly affect an individual's longevity and health. In China, the environment has long been considered an important factor in the longevity of the population.

In many areas of China, life has always been very active, with a strong emphasis on the outdoors and being in contact with nature.

China is also known for its walking culture, which encourages taking long walks in the fresh air and walking on a regular basis.

Furthermore, rural areas in China are often equipped with sources of clean and fresh water, which are considered essential for health and longevity.

The quality of the air we breathe is also a very important factor. In fact, in many rural areas of China, the air is cleaner and free of pollutants than in large ones city and this helps maintain lung health and therefore allows you to live longer.

Chapter 13

The power of Kung Fu: the ancient Chinese martial art for physical and mental strength

Kung Fu is a Chinese martial art that has ancient roots dating back to at least the Song Dynasty period. The word "Kung Fu" means literally "to work hard" or "master of work", and refers to the skill of practicing a martial art with commitment, determination and skill.

Kung Fu encompasses a wide range of styles and techniques, including Wing Chun, Shaolin and Tai Chi Chuan, and is used to improve physical, mental and spiritual health. Kung Fu practice also includes breathing techniques, meditation and concentration, and aiming to develop a balance between mind, body and spirit.

Kung Fu is a martial art that has developed in the context of society

China and its cultural traditions. The practice of Kung Fu has been influenced by Taoist, Buddhist and Confucian philosophies, and is still practiced as a form of self-defense and as a means to improve health and well-being.

It is also a social practice that is often practiced in groups. This type of social interaction can be especially helpful for young people trying to develop a sense of identity and community. Furthermore, the practice of Kung Fu in a group can be a way to build stronger interpersonal relationships and increase self-confidence.

Kung Fu is a martial art that is passed down from generation to generation, and therefore represents one cultural tradition that is preserved and preserved.

This tradition continues to be an important part of Chinese culture and a way to connect with one's history and cultural roots.

Furthermore, Kung Fu is not only a martial art, but also a form of artistic expression. The practice of Kung Fu also includes performing martial arts performances, which are a popular form of entertainment in China and abroad.

Worldwide. These shows include acrobatics and martial skill demonstrations, and often feature traditional Chinese stories or legends.

The practice of this discipline is not limited only to an elite of people but can be practiced by people of all ages, genders and physical abilities. There are many Kung Fu schools and teachers offering courses for all levels, from beginners to advanced. Kung Fu practice can be tailored to meet each practitioner's individual needs, regardless of their age, health or physical abilities.

It increases flexibility, strength and endurance, improves posture and coordination, and can help prevent injuries. Also, practicing breathing and meditation techniques can
help reduce stress and improve mental health.

If you have come this far, it means that you have really understood that there is something to change in your life, which does not allow you to achieve the desired results or simply you are enjoying this reading; in both cases, thank you and ask you to continue.

Get inspired by this guide to start DOING better and GIVE your best: at the table, in the gym and in general in your life.

Conclusion

The Chinese cultural tradition represents an invaluable wealth for humanity.

With a history dating back over 5,000 years, Chinese culture has developed many practices that have allowed it's inhabitants to live long and healthy lives. These practices include a balanced diet based on the Yin and Yang philosophy, the use of traditional medicine techniques such as Acupuncture, Moxibustion and Tui Na massage, practice of martial arts such as Tai Chi, Qigong and Kung Fu, and many other cultural traditions that have been passed down from generation to generation.

In this book we have explored these aspects of Chinese culture in depth and seen how closely they are interconnected and yes influence each other. We have also seen how these practices have been used to maintain the health and longevity of the Chinese for centuries.

Chinese culture represents a treasure trove of knowledge and wisdom that it is still very current and relevant to the daily lives of many Chinese people and people from all over the world. It's important so continue to explore and appreciate these traditions, not only for their history and beauty, but also for their myriad health and well-being benefits.

The Chinese cultural tradition has been a source of inspiration for many other cultures around the world. The Chinese philosophy of Taoism, for example, has influenced many religions and philosophies, not only in China but also in other parts of the world. This philosophy emphasizes the importance of balance and harmony with nature, and this has been a major theme in Chinese culture for centuries.

Balanced nutrition based on the philosophy of Yin and Yang is another practice that has had a significant impact on Chinese culture. This philosophy holds that each food has unique properties that affect the body and mind different way. For example, hot foods like chili peppers are considered Yang, while cold foods like ice cream are considered Yin. The Yin and Yang philosophy encourages eating a balanced diet that includes both hot and cold foods to keep the body in balance.

Traditional Chinese medicine is another practice that has had a significant impact on Chinese culture. This medicine uses techniques such as acupuncture, moxibustion and tui na massage to treat a variety of ailments and diseases. These techniques are still very popular in China and many others parts of the world, and many studies have demonstrated their effectiveness in treating many health conditions.

Martial arts such as Tai Chi, Qigong and Kung Fu have been practiced in China for centuries and are still very popular today. These martial arts are not only a way to maintain physical fitness and health, but also a way to improve concentration, calmness and mental discipline.

Ultimately, the Chinese cultural tradition represents a wealth invaluable to mankind, and continue to explore and appreciate these traditions is important not only for their history and beauty, but also for the many benefits they have on health and well-being. Chinese culture represents a treasure trove of knowledge and wisdom that will continue to inspire and influence the world for many generations to come, and I sincerely hope it inspires you too, thanks to this guide.

Thanks for reading.

Jean-Claude Marchetti

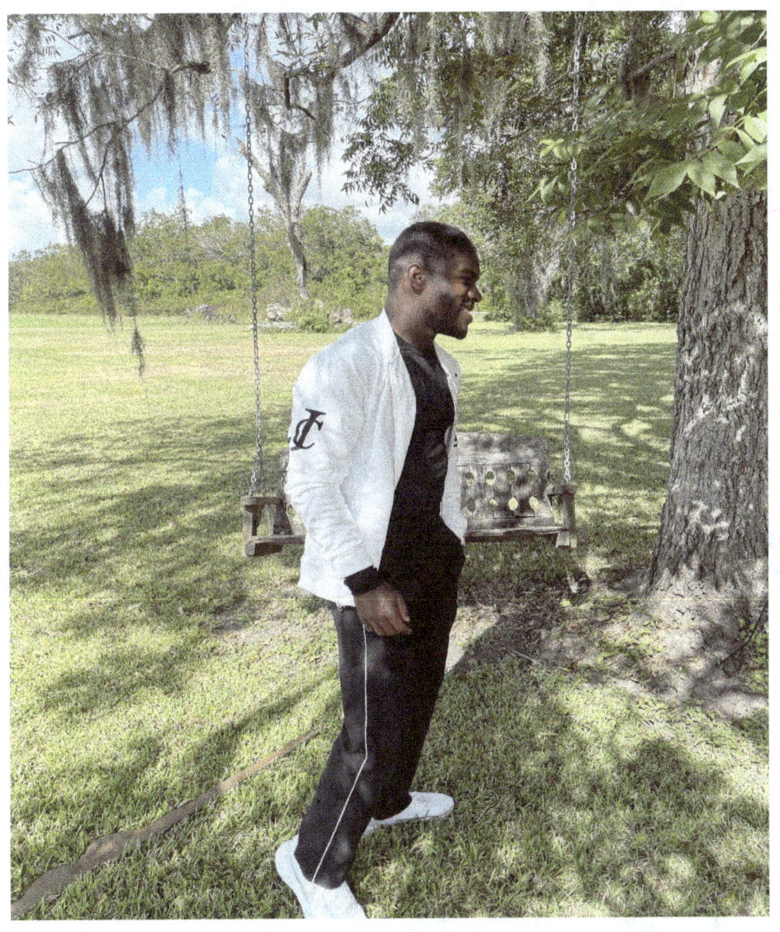